61 Organic Meal Recipes to Help Prevent Cancer:

Naturally Strengthen and Boost Your Immune System to Fight Cancer

By

Joe Correa CSN

COPYRIGHT

ACKNOWLEDGEMENTS

This book is dedicated to my friends and family that have had mild or serious illnesses so that you may find a solution and make the necessary changes in your life.

61 Organic Meal Recipes to Help Prevent Cancer:

Naturally Strengthen and Boost Your Immune System to Fight Cancer

By

Joe Correa CSN

CONTENTS

ABOUT THE AUTHOR

After years of Research, I honestly believe in the positive effects that proper nutrition can have over the body and mind. My knowledge and experience has helped me live healthier throughout the years and which I have shared with family and friends. The more you know about eating and drinking healthier, the sooner you will want to change your life and eating habits.

Nutrition is a key part in the process of being healthy and living longer so get started today. The first step is the most important and the most significant.

INTRODUCTION

61 Organic Meal Recipes to Help Prevent Cancer: Naturally Strengthen and Boost Your Immune System to Fight Cancer

By Joe Correa CSN

Cancer is a disease that takes millions of lives every year, and it can come at ano matter what your age. It also affects people who live completely healthy lives. However, the best thing you can do is to be as informed as possible about how to prevent this terrible disease.

Studies show that 33% of all types of cancer can be prevented with a healthy lifestyle. But, this is primarily related to healthy eating and physical activity.

In this book, we have prepared the finest selection of recipes with ingredients recommended by experts, as the best way to prevent cancer.

Fresh fruits, various types of vegetables rich in fiber, reduced salt intake, are some of the most important things you need to focus on when changing your diet.

These recipes will help you reach a healthy weight which should also be your ideal weight since this is also an important factor when trying to live a healthy cancer-free lifestyle. Obesity is associated with a higher risk of cancer.

Quitting or reducing alcohol consumption and quit smoking will help your immune system to be stronger so that it can fight any disease.

These recipes use the most potent ingredients against cancer. For example, a tomato is great for prostate cancer, white and red onions will protect your stomach, colon, and rectum, while Vitamin C is magnificent for the esophagus.

Vitamins and minerals can be taken through supplements, but it is always recommended to go straight to the source which would be from fruits and vegetables. These recipes contain hundreds of other phytonutrients that can't be found in multivitamin tablets. Some of these substances are: flavonoids (from citrus fruits, berries, etc.), various pigments with antioxidants (from grapes, eggplant, red cabbage), quercetin (from apple, onion,) carotenoids (from carrots, melons, apricots), lycopene (from tomatoes), lutein for eye (from spinach and kale).

Make a change for good!

61 ORGANIC MEAL RECIPES TO HELP PREVENT CANCER: NATURALLY STRENGTHEN AND BOOST YOUR IMMUNE SYSTEM TO FIGHT CANCER

Breakfast Recipes

1. Banana Manuka honey smoothie

Ingredients:

1 cup of chilled apple juice

Handful of chopped spinach

1 banana, medium-sized

2 tsp of Manuka honey

grated ginger, to taste

Preparation:

Toss all the ingredients into your blender and turn it on. Keep blending till the banana and spinach are completely smooth. Your Manuka honey smoothie is ready!

Nutrition information per serving: Kcal: 238 Protein: 7.5g, Carbs: 35g, Fats: 5g

2. Apple muesli with goji berries and flax seeds

Ingredients:

1 cup rolled oats

½ cup dried goji berries

2 large apples

3 tablespoons Flax Seeds

3 tablespoons honey

1 ¼ cups coconut water

1 ¼ cups plain yogurt

2 tablespoons mint leaves

Himalayan crystal salt, to taste

Preparation:

Grate the apples into a large bowl. Put the yogurt, Goji berries, flax seeds, rolled oats, mint and coconut water in the bowl and mix well. Leave the mixture in the fridge overnight. Blend the salt and honey into the muesli and serve!

Nutrition information per serving: Kcal: 280 Protein: 4g, Carbs: 44.5, Fats: 6g

3. Organic Deli burrito with spinach

Ingredients

2 slices of organic deli meat

1 teaspoon of ghee

2 whole eggs

¼ cup of chopped spinach

Pinch of salt

2 tablespoons of minced bell pepper

1 small tomato, minced

Guacamole sauce and Fresh cilantro, for serving

Preparation:

Whisk the eggs and salt in a mixing bowl and set aside. In a pan, apply medium-high heat and add the ghee. Sauté the spinach, tomato and bell pepper for 3 minutes. Add the eggs and scramble the mixture with a spatula. When the scrambled egg is done, remove from heat and add into each sliced deli meat.

Roll the ham and secure the end with a toothpick. Brown the deli meat evenly on all sides and transfer to a serving plate. Serve warm with guacamole and cilantro.

Nutrition information per serving: Kcal: 300 Protein: 19g, Carbs: 75.5g, Fats: 20g

4. Cashews Porridge

Ingredients:

1 ripe yellow banana, sliced

2 cups of unsweetened coconut milk

½ tablespoon of cinnamon

½ cup chopped cashews

½ cup chopped almonds

½ cup chopped pecans

Pinch of salt

Preparation:

In a mixing bowl, place the nuts and pour in with just enough water to cover. Sprinkle with salt, cover bowl and soak overnight. Drain and rinse with running water. Transfer into a food processor together with the banana, coconut milk, and cinnamon. Process the ingredients until thick and smooth.

Place the mixture in a pan over medium-high heat. Cook for about 5 minutes, or until it reaches to a boil while stirring regularly. Portion into 4 individual serving bowls and serve with extra chopped nuts if desired.

Nutrition information per serving: Kcal: 300 Protein: 7.2g, Carbs: 17.5g, Fats: 25.5g

5. Cherry tomato omelet

Ingredients:

4 medium free-range whole eggs, beaten

½ cup cottage cheese

½ cup diced white onion

1 cup fresh spinach

6 pieces of cherry tomatoes, diced

1 tablespoon of olive oil

Salt and pepper, to taste

Preparation:

Add the oil in a skillet and apply with medium heat. Sauté the onions until soft and pour in the beaten eggs. Cook for about 3 minutes or until the bottom part is lightly brown.

Add the cheese, spinach and tomatoes on one side of the egg and season to taste with salt and pepper. Carefully lift the other side of the omelet and flip it over to cover the vegetables. Reduce the heat to low and cook for about 2 minutes.

Slide the omelet onto a serving plate and serve with extra cheese on top.

Nutrition information per serving: Kcal: 140 Protein: 14g, Carbs: 3.5g, Fats: 8.5g

6. Almond meal pancakes

Ingredients:

1 cup almond flour

2 medium free-range whole eggs

½ cup water

½ teaspoon baking soda

¼ teaspoon salt

¼ teaspoon of sugar

2 ounces of ghee

Directions:

Combine together the flour, salt and baking soda in a mixing bowl and set aside. In a separate bowl, whisk together the eggs, sugar and 1 tablespoon of ghee until well combined. Pour the egg mixture into the bowl with the flour mixture and mix it thoroughly until smooth. If the batter mixture is too thick, add water and mix until the desired consistency is achieved. Cover the bowl with a cloth and let it sit for 15 minutes, set aside.

Add the remaining ghee into a pan and apply with medium-high heat. Once the ghee is hot, pour in enough pancake mixture just to cover the base of the pan. Cook until the bottom part is lightly browned and flip it over to cook the other side. Repeat the procedure with the remaining pancake mixture and place them on a serving platter.

Serve warm with your favorite spread, if desired.

Nutrition information per serving: Kcal: 149 Protein: 6.1g, Carbs: 4g, Fats: 13,5g

7. Shredded Coconut Blackberry Pudding with Chia and Pistachios

Ingredients:

1 cup of almond milk

½ teaspoon of almond extract

½ cup of crushed fresh blackberries

3 tablespoons of chia seeds

1 tablespoon of shredded coconut

¼ cup of chopped raw pistachios

Preparation:

Combine together the crushed blackberries, chia seeds, almond extract, almond milk and shredded coconut in a mixing bowl. Mix the ingredients well until well combined.

Cover the bowl with plastic wrap and refrigerate for at least 12 hours before serving.

Serve the blackberry pudding with chopped pistachios on top.

Nutrition information per serving: Kcal: 300 Protein: 19g, Carbs: 50.5g, Fats: 6.5g

8. Blueberry Breakfast Tortilla

Ingredients:

1 tablespoon of extra virgin olive oil

4 eggs, beaten

1 tablespoon of almond butter

Pinch of black pepper

1 teaspoon of ground cinnamon

½ cup of fresh blueberries

Preparation:

Whisk together the almond butter, eggs, cinnamon and pepper in a bowl and set aside.

In a skillet, apply medium heat and add the oil. Pour in the egg mixture and cook for 3 minutes without stirring. Top with blueberries and cover with lid. Reduce to low heat and cook for 6 to 8 minutes more.

Remove the lid, place a plate on top of the skillet and flip the skillet to remove the egg tortilla. Return the skillet to the stove, slide in the tortilla in the skillet to cook the other side. Cover and cook for 3 to 4 minutes more.

When the blueberry tortilla is done, slide into a serving plate and serve warm.

Nutrition information per serving: Kcal: 168 Protein: 6g, Carbs: 24.5g, Fats: 6g

9. Buckwheat with cranberries

Ingredients:

1 cup of fresh cranberries

1 cups of buckwheat groats

1 medium apple, peeled and cut into slices

1 cup of low - fat yogurt

3 egg whites

½ cup of maple syrup

Preparation:

Preheat the oven to 350 degrees. Spread the buckwheat groats over a baking sheet and toast for about 5-6 minutes. You want a nice lightly brown color.

Boil the cranberries over a high temperature. Cook until they burst. Add the toasted buckwheat groats, egg whites, and apple slices and stir well. Cook for another 7 minutes, or until the buckwheat groats are cooked. Stir in the maple syrup. Remove from the heat and let it stand for 10 minutes. Serve cold topped with yogurt.

Nutrition information per serving: Kcal: 158 Protein: 4g, Carbs: 22.5g, Fats: 4.5g

10. Apple and quinoa muesli with walnuts

Ingredients:

½ cup of ground walnuts

2 large apples

3 tbsp of flax seeds

3 tbsp of brown sugar

1 ¼ cups of coconut water

1 ¼ cups of yogurt

1 cup of quinoa

2 tablespoons of mint leaves

Preparation:

Wash and peel the apples. Cut them into bite - size pieces and place in a large bowl. Add yogurt, walnuts, flax seeds, quinoa seeds, mint and coconut water in the bowl and stir well. Leave the mixture in the fridge overnight.

Top with honey before serving.

Nutrition information per serving: Kcal: 215 Protein: 8.3g, Carbs: 24.4g, Fats: 10.5g

11. Frozen cream with blueberries

Ingredients:

1 cup of low fat cream

1 cup of fresh blueberries

¼ cup of skim milk

2 egg whites

1 tbsp of honey

1 tsp of brown sugar

Preparation:

Combine the ingredients in a large bowl. Beat well with a fork. Put it in a freezer for about 30 minutes. This creamy mixture goes perfectly with a gluten-free, buckwheat toast.

Nutrition information per serving: Kcal: 101 Protein: 2.5g, Carbs: 19.5g, Fats: 0g

12. Peanut butter oats

Ingredients:

1 cup of oats, cooked

1 cup of unsweetened almond milk

2 tbsp of organic peanut butter

1 tbsp of strawberry syrup

1 tsp of cinnamon

Preparation:

Place the ingredients in a bowl and stir well until you get a nice, smooth mixture. If necessary, add some water. Pour this mixture in a tall glasses and leave in the refrigerator overnight.

13. Egg and cheese sandwich with dry parsley

Ingredients:

4 eggs

1 cup of cottage cheese

1 tsp of dried parsley

8 thin slices of whole grain bread

salt to taste

Preparation:

Boil the eggs for 10 minutes. Allow to cool and peel them. Cut into thin slices – about 5-6 slices of each egg. Layer 1 tbsp of low-fat cottage cheese on top of the bread and top with the egg, sliced.

Nutrition information per serving: Kcal: 280 Protein: 14g, Carbs: 27g, Fats: 13g

14. Fried egg whites with cottage cheese

Ingredients:

4 eggs

1 cup of cottage cheese

¼ cup of skim milk

1 tbsp of olive oil

salt to taste

Preparation:

Remove the egg whites from yolks. Grease the frying pan with olive oil. Heat up over to medium-high heat. Whisk together egg whites, cottage cheese, and milk. Add some salt to taste. Fry for 3-4 minutes, stirring constantly.

Nutrition information per serving: Kcal: 360 Protein: 34g, Carbs: 12.5g, Fats: 17.5g

15. Feta and eggs toast

Ingredients:

4 slices of whole grain bread

3 eggs

1 cup of baby spinach, chopped

½ cup of feta cheese

2 tbsp of extra virgin olive oil

Preparation:

Beat the eggs with a fork in a bowl. Cut feta cheese into small cubes and add them to the bowl. Grease the frying pan with olive oil. Heat up over to medium-high heat and fry baby spinach for several minutes, stirring constantly. Add egg and feta mixture and fry for several more minutes.

Put the bread in the toaster for 2 minutes. Serve with egg, feta and spinach mixture.

Nutrition information per serving: Kcal: 317 Protein: 15.5g, Carbs: 20.5g, Fats: 19.5g

16. Spinach omelet

Ingredients:

4 eggs

1 cup of baby spinach leaves, chopped

1 tbsp of onion powder

¼ tsp of ground red pepper

¼ tsp of sea salt

1 tbsp of Parmesan cheese

1 tbsp of olive oil

Preparation:

Beat the eggs with a fork, in a large bowl. Add baby spinach and Parmesan cheese. Mix well. Season with onion powder, red pepper and sea salt.

Heat upIn a bowl, beat the eggs, and stir in the baby spinach and Parmesan cheese. Season with onion powder, nutmeg, salt, and pepper.

Heat up the olive oil over a medium heat. Add egg mixture and fry for 2-3 minutes.

Nutrition information per serving: Kcal: 215 Protein: 24g, Carbs: 3g, Fats: 14g

17. Quinoa cereal

Ingredients:

1 cup of quinoa cereal

1 cup of plums, cut in half and pitted

1 tbsp of sugar

2 tbsp of maple syrup

1 tbsp of coconut oil, melted

½ tsp of cinnamon, ground

1 tsp of vanilla extract

water

Preparation:

Put your plums in a large skillet and add enough water to cover them. Bring it to boil and cook for 10 minutes, or until tender. Remove from the heat and drain. Set aside.

Use the same skillet to boil 2 cups of water. Add quinoa cereals, sugar, maple syrup, coconut oil, cinnamon, and vanilla extract. Reduce the heat to minimum and cook until slightly thickened. This should take about 5 minutes.

Remove from the heat and pour into bowls. Top with plums.

Nutrition information per serving: Kcal: 131 Protein: 4.4g, Carbs: 23g, Fats: 3g

18. Coconut bananas

Ingredients:

2 large bananas, sliced lengthwise

1 cup of coconut milk

1 tsp of coconut oil

1 tsp of coconut extract

2 tbsp of agave syrup

¼ tsp of cinnamon

Preparation:

Pour 1 cup of coconut milk in a small saucepan. Bring it to boil and stir in coconut oil, coconut extract, and agave syrup. Cook for one minute and remove from the heat. Allow it to cool for a while.

Pour this mixture on each banana slice and sprinkle with some cinnamon. Serve cold.

Nutrition information per serving: Kcal: 182 Protein: 2.6g, Carbs: 28.8g, Fats: 7.3g

19. Eggplant French toast

Ingredients:

1 large eggplant

3 eggs

¼ tsp of sea salt

1 tbsp of oil

½ tsp of cinnamon

Preparation:

Peel eggplant and cut lengthwise into slices. Sprinkle salt on each side of eggplant. Allow it to rest for few minutes. Rinse well and press gently to drain and extract any excess liquid.

Meanwhile, mix eggs with cinnamon in a large bowl. Heat up 1 tbsp of oil in frying pan over a high temperature.

Put your eggplant slices in egg mixture. Make few holes with a knife to allow the mixture to permeate the eggplant. Fry it until golden brown color, on each side. Serve your 'French toast' warm.

Nutrition information per serving: Kcal: 118 Protein: 4g, Carbs: 12g, Fats: 8g

20. Cottage cheese and banana pancakes

Ingredients:

1 cup of sliced banana

½ cup of rice fluor

½ cup of skim milk

½ cup of almond milk

3 tbsp of brown sugar

1 tsp of vanilla extract

1 egg

½ cup of low fat cream

non-fat cooking spray

Preparation:

Combine banana slices, rice flour, skim milk and almond milk in a bowl and mix with an electric mixer until smooth mixture. Cover it and let it stand for 15 minutes.

In another bowl, mix the cream with sugar vanilla extract and egg. Beat well with a fork, or even better with an electric mixer. You want to get a foamy mixture. Set aside.

Sprinkle some non-fat cooking spray on a frying pan. Use ¼ cup of banana mixture to make one pancake. Fry your pancakes for about 2-3 minutes on each side. This mixture should give you 8 pancakes.

Spread 1 tbsp of cheese mixture over each pancake and serve.

Nutrition information per serving: Kcal: 340 Protein: 22g, Carbs: 42g, Fats: 8.5g

Lunch Recipes

21. Ginger and chili chicken thighs

Ingredients:

2 pounds chicken thighs (skin and bone should be left on)

1 tablespoon chili powder

Fresh basil

Black pepper, freshly ground

Sea salt

16 ounces coconut water

1 tablespoon grated ginger, fresh

1 tablespoon coriander seeds

8 peeled and lightly smashed garlic cloves

Preparation:

Put the chicken thighs along with garlic in the slow cooker. Add rest of the spices, sprinkling them evenly over the chicken thighs. Pour the coconut water on the thighs and add the fresh basil. Cover the slow cooker and set the heat to low. You need to cook the thighs for around 8 to 10 hours before they are tender enough to eat. The liquid will also give off an enticing aroma when the ginger chili chicken is ready.

Nutrition information per serving: Kcal: 262 Protein: 26.6g, Carbs: 17.4g, Fats: 8g

22. Beef stew

Ingredients:

2 pounds grass-fed stew beef

1 tablespoon flax seed oil

6 ounces tomato paste

2 handfuls baby carrots

2 quartered sweet potatoes

1 chopped large yellow onion

1 handful fresh mushrooms

½ tablespoon salt

1 bay leaf

2 ½ cups beef broth

½ cup frozen green peas

1 teaspoon thyme

3 minced garlic cloves

Preparation:

Take a frying pan and set it over high heat. Heat up the oil and add the beef to it. Fry the beef on all sides until properly brown. You may have to use more oil depending on how long it takes for a side to brown. Once the beef is brown, transfer it to the slow cooker. In the same pan, fry the onions, turning the heat to medium. Cook the onions for around 5 minutes.

Pour about ½ cup of water and the tomato paste in the frying pan to scoop up any remaining bits of the beef and onions. After this, pour the mixture over the beef in a deep pot. Put in all the remaining ingredients and stir properly, especially if the liquid is thick. Cover the pot, set the heat to low and cook for about an hour. 15 minutes before taking it off, toss in the frozen green peas to give them enough time to melt and cook.

Nutrition information per serving: Kcal: 220 Protein: 12g, Carbs: 16g, Fats: 13.2g

23. Chili Stew

Ingredients:

1 pound ground beef

8 minced garlic cloves

1 teaspoon garlic powder

2 tablespoons olive oil

1 tablespoon cumin

3 tablespoons chili powder

2 cups sliced mushrooms

1 pound cubed stew beef

1 chopped medium zucchini

1 minced medium onion

28 ounces tomato sauce

½ cup pureed carrots

2 cups beef broth

Preparation:

Put the ground beef in a frying pan along with a little oil. Set the heat to high and fry till the beef turns brown on all sides. Once browned, transfer the beef to the slow cooker. In the slow cooker, add the cumin, carrots, chili powder, beef broth, tomato sauce and garlic powder to the ground beef. Stir properly to mix the ingredients in.

Use the frying pan to sauté the onion, mushrooms, zucchini, and garlic. The purpose is to soften each vegetable. Move the vegetables from the frying pan to the slow cooker once soft. Place the stew beef in the pan along with olive oil and chili powder. Fry till the beef turns brown on all sides and then move to crock pot. Cover the slow cooker, turn the heat to low and cook for 5 to 8 hours.

Nutrition information per serving: Kcal: 170 Protein: 7g, Carbs: 21.7g, Fats: 6.6g

24. Nacho casserole

Ingredients:

1 pound of ground beef

1 small onion, peeled and chopped

1 cup of spicy red beans

½ cup of canned corn, cooked

½ cup of sugar-free tomato sauce

2 tbsp of taco seasoning mix

1 cup of cottage cheese

1 cup of chopped green onions

Preparation:

Cook ground beef over a medium-high temperature, stirring occasionally. This process should take about 30 minutes. Remove from heat and drain well. Cut into bite size pieces and combine with red beans, corn, tomato sauce and seasoning mix. Stir well and simmer over medium heat for about 10 minutes.

Preheat oven to 350 degrees. Pour half of this mixture into baking casserole pan. Top with cottage cheese and green onions and add the remaining beef mixture. Bake for about 25 minutes.

Nutrition information per serving: Kcal: 450 Protein: 32.8g, Carbs: 18.4g, Fats: 29g

25. Striped bass

Ingredients:

4 large striped bass

1 tablespoon olive oil

½ tsp of sea salt

¼ tsp of black pepper

1 cup cottage cheese

Preparation:

Combine oil salt and pepper. Use a kitchen brush to spread this mixture over fish. Grill fish over a medium-high temperature, on each side for about 5 minutes. Serve with cottage cheese.

Nutrition information per serving: Kcal: 154 Protein: 28g, Carbs: 5g, Fats: 8.3g

26. Green chicken

Ingredients:

3 pieces of chicken breast (about 1 pound)

2 cups of spinach, chopped

1 cup of low - fat yogurt

3 green peppers

3 chili peppers

2 small onions, chopped

1 tbsp of ground ginger

1 tsp of red pepper powder

4 tbsp of oil

salt to taste

Preparation:

Wash and pat dry the chicken using a kitchen paper. Chop into bite size pieces. Finely chop onion and peppers and set aside.

Heat up the oil in a large weasel. Add onions and peppers and sauté for few minutes. Now add chicken breast pieces, ground ginger, red pepper powder, and salt. Stir-fry for ten minutes, or until the chicken turns light brown.

Meanwhile, combine low fat yogurt with spinach in a food processor. Mix well for 30 seconds. Add this mixture to the weasel and fry until the spinach gets well mashed. Cover the weasel, remove from the heat and let it stand for about 10 minutes before serving.

Nutrition information per serving: Kcal: 380 Protein: 16g, Carbs: 54.5g, Fats: 12g

27. Chicken in mushroom sauce

Ingredients:

1 pound of chicken meat, skinless

2 tbsp of all - purpose flour

1 cup of button mushrooms

1 cup of green beans, cooked

¼ cup of chicken broth

½ tsp of sea salt

¼ tsp of black pepper

4 tbsp of olive oil

Preparation:

Wash and pat dry the chicken meat. In a large bowl, combine all - purpose flour with salt and pepper. Coat the chicken with the flour and set aside. Heat up the olive oil over a medium temperature and fry chicken meat for about 5 minutes on each side. Remove from the saucepan and transfer to a plate. In the same saucepan add chicken broth, green beans, and button mushrooms. Bring it to a boil and cook for 2-3 minutes. Return the chicken and cook for another 20 minutes, stirring occasionally, until the water evaporates. Serve warm.

Nutrition information per serving: Kcal: 290 Protein: 21g, Carbs: 36g, Fats: 7g

28. Red beans mix

Ingredients:

1 cup of red beans, canned and cooked

½ cup of green beans

½ cup of button mushrooms

1 cup of cottage cheese

1 cup of Greek yogurt

2 egg whites

2 tbsp of coconut oil

1 tsp of sea salt

Preparation:

Combine the ingredients in a food processor. Mix well for 30 seconds. Preheat the oven to 300 degrees. Coat the small baking dish with 2 tbsp of olive oil. Pour the red beans mixture in a baking dish and bake for about 10-15 minutes. You want to get a nice light brown color. Remove from the oven, let it stand for about 10 minutes and cut into 4 equal pieces. Serve warm.

Nutrition information per serving: Kcal: 193 Protein: 5.4g, Carbs: 23.6g, Fats: 10.2g

29. Greek style chicken

Ingredients:

4 pieces of chicken breast halves

1 cup of cottage cheese

½ cup of Greek yogurt

1 cup of chopped cucumber

1 cup of chopped lettuce

1 cup of cherry tomatoes

½ cup of chopped onions

5 garlic cloves

2 tbsp of fresh lemon juice

1 tbsp of dried oregano

½ tsp of red pepper

½ tsp of salt

2 tbsp of olive oil

6 whole-wheat pitas, cut into wedges

Preparation:

Wash and cut the meat into small pieces. Set aside.

Combine the cottage cheese, Greek yogurt, vegetables and spices in a food processor. Mix well for 30 seconds. Heat up the olive oil over a medium temperature. Fry chicken chops for about 20 minutes, stirring constantly. Add the vegetable mixture to the saucepan. Stir well and cook for another 10 minutes. Remove from the heat and shape this mixture into 6 equal parts. Serve with pitas.

Nutrition information per serving: Kcal: 498 Protein: 23.6g, Carbs: 23.5g, Fats: 24

30. Cottage cheese with fried vegetables

Ingredients:

½ cup of cottage cheese

1 small onion

1 small carrot

1 small tomato

2 medium red peppers

salt to taste

1 tbsp of olive oil

Preparation:

Wash and pat dry the vegetables using a kitchen paper. Cut into thin slices or strips. Heat up the olive oil over a medium temperature and fry the vegetables for about 10 minutes, stirring constantly. Add salt and mix well. You want to wait until the vegetables soften, then add cottage cheese. Stir well. Fry for another 2-3 minutes. Remove from the heat and serve.

Nutrition information per serving: Kcal: 122 Protein: 11.5g, Carbs: 8.5g, Fats: 5.5g

31. Green bean burritos

Ingredients:

1 cup of cooked green beans

1 pound of lean veal, chopped

1 cup of Cheddar

½ cup of chopped onions

1 tsp of ground red pepper

1 tsp of chili powder

6 whole grain tortillas

Preparation:

Combine the meat with ground red pepper, chili powder, and onions in a frying pan. Stir well for 15 minutes on a low temperature. Remove from the heat.

Mix Cheddar with green beans in a blender. Mix well for about 30 seconds. Add the cheese mixture to the meat. Divide this mixture into 6 equal pieces and spread over tortillas. Wrap and serve.

Nutrition information per serving: Kcal: 370 Protein: 15 g, Carbs: 55.5g, Fats: 11g

32. Roasted lentils

Ingredients:

½ cups of uncooked lentils

1 tbsp of salt

2 tbsp of olive oil

1 tsp of pepper

1 tsp of red chili powder

1 tsp of cinnamon powder

Preparation:

First, you want to cook lentils. Pour about 2 cups of water in a saucepan and bring it to boil. Add lentils and boil for about 15-20 minutes, until soft from inside and still hold their shape. Remove from the heat and rinse well with cold water. Drain your chia seeds and set aside.

Preheat the oven to 300 degrees. In a large bowl, coat the lentils with salt, olive oil, pepper, red chili powder and cinnamon. Spread the lentils over a medium sized baking dish and bake for about 20 minutes.

Prepared like this, lentils can be stored in the airtight container for about 15 days.

Nutrition information per serving: Kcal: 110 Protein: 8g, Carbs: 19g, Fats: 3.5g

33. Seafood Balls

Ingredients:

1½ pounds white fish

Sea salt

Black pepper, freshly ground

½ pound shrimp

½ lemon juice

1½ cups almond flour

2 tablespoons tartar sauce

½ cup water

3 tablespoons fresh parsley

3 eggs

Cooking fat

Preparation:

Use a food processor to make a paste combining 2 eggs, ½ cup almond flour, shrimps, white fish, parsley, and lemon juice, blending till the paste is smooth. Take a bowl, pour some water and break an egg into it. Whisk the two and create a mixture. In a separate bowl, put the remaining almond flour and add salt and pepper to it.

Take a larger bowl and mix the contents of all three bowls. Then, make small balls out of the batter you have created. Put the balls in the skillet and fry for about 15 minutes. Enjoy with tartar sauce.

Nutrition information per serving: Kcal: 101 Protein: 9.4g, Carbs: 10.2g, Fats: 3.7g

34. Cayenne Pepper Shrimps

Ingredients:

2 pounds peeled and deveined large shrimps

2 tablespoons lemon juice

Cayenne pepper

Black pepper

Sea salt

4 minced garlic cloves

3 tablespoons butter

2 tablespoons chopped fresh parsley

2 tablespoons cooking fat

Preparation:

Take a frying pan and put in the butter. Heat until the butter melts and then throw in the shrimps. Fry the shrimps till almost opaque in appearance. Move shrimps to the large pan and fry the garlic for a minute or two. Add the rest of the ingredients, along with the garlic, to the pan. Cover and cook for 20 minutes over a medium temperature.

Nutrition information per serving: Kcal: 162 Protein: 24.6g, Carbs: 1.7g, Fats: 6.2g

35. Warm chicken bowl

Ingredients:

28 ounces diced fire roasted tomatoes

12 boneless & skinless chicken thighs

1 tablespoon dried basil

8 ounces full - fat coconut milk

Salt & pepper

7 ounces tomato paste

3 chopped celery stalks

3 chopped carrots

2 tablespoons coconut oil

1 finely chopped onion

4 minced garlic cloves

½ container mushrooms

Preparation:

Pour coconut oil in a frying pan and put over high heat. Add the celery, onions, and carrots and fry for 5 to 10 minutes. Move them to the skillet and add tomato paste, basil, garlic, mushrooms and seasoning. Keep stirring the vegetables till they are completely covered by tomato sauce. At the same time, cut the chicken into small cubes to make it easier to eat.

Put the chicken in the skillet, pour the coconut oil over it and throw in the tomatoes. Stir the chicken in to ensure the ingredients and vegetables are properly mixed with it. Turn the heat to low and cook for about 30 minutes. The vegetables and chicken should be cooked through before you turn the heat off. Pour some coconut milk on top before serving!

Nutrition information per serving: Kcal: 189 Protein: 4.2g, Carbs: 25.1g, Fats: 8g

36. Autumn Soup

Ingredients:

3 sliced sweet potatoes

Salt

vanilla extract

2 sliced fennel bulbs

15 ounces pureed pumpkin

1 large onion sliced

coconut oil

pumpkin pie spice

50 ounces boiling water

Preparation:

In the crock pot, melt around 1 tablespoon of oil on high heat. Then, turn the heat to low and put in onion and fennel bulbs. Continue cooking till they are caramelized. Add the rest of the ingredients to the pot and continue cooking till the sweet potatoes are sour. Cook on low heat to get the best possible result. After the process is completed, blend the soup until it is smooth and then add salt to taste.

Nutrition information per serving: Kcal: 115 Protein: 8.2g, Carbs: 14.3g, Fats: 3.2g

37. Spanish chicken

Ingredients:

6 chicken thighs

Half a cauliflower head

salt

1 can of chopped tomatoes

½ pound Brussels sprouts

1 medium chorizo sausage

3 medium zucchinis

Preparation:

Take a frying pan and add some oil. Fry the chicken thighs, removing the skin if you want, until they turn golden brown. Remove the thighs from the frying pan and move to a large pot. Next, chop the sausage and fry for around 3 minutes. After frying, put it in the pot as well.

Slice the zucchinis and break the cauliflower into small florets and put them in the pot as well. Also, add the Brussels sprouts to the pot. Add salt and then pour the chopped tomatoes over the ingredients. Set the heat to low and cook for about an hour. Serve with a side of baby corn.

Nutrition information per serving: Kcal: 430 Protein: 34.8g, Carbs: 39.5g, Fats: 15g

38. Onion-mushrooms beef tips

Ingredients:

2 pounds of grass-fed beef stew meat, cubed

Salt and ground pepper, to taste

2 tablespoons of olive oil

2 cups of fresh white mushrooms

2 cups of beef stock

½ white onion, chopped

1 tablespoon minced garlic

Preparation:

Season the beef with salt and pepper and toss to coat it evenly with spices.

In a stew pot over medium-high heat, add the oil and brown the beef evenly on all sides. Stir in the garlic and onions, sauté for 2 minutes and add the mushrooms

Add the oil in the inner pot, press the sauté button and adjust to brown mode. Season beef with salt and pepper and brown evenly on all sides in the inner pot. Stir in the onions and garlic and sauté for about 1 minute and then add the mushrooms and the stock. Cover with lid, bring it to a boil and reduce to low heat. Simmer for about 30 minutes or until the meat is tender and cooked through.

Adjust the seasoning and transfer into a serving bowl. Serve immediately.

Nutrition information per serving: Kcal: 158 Protein: 18.8g, Carbs: 2.7g, Fats: 8g

39. Turkey in orange sauce

Ingredients:

2 tablespoons of extra virgin olive oil

1 pound of turkey breast slices

Salt and ground black pepper, to taste

1 cup of chicken stock

2 tablespoons of olive oil, for the sauce

2 packets of sugar

2 teaspoons grated orange zest

2 tablespoons of fresh orange, juiced

1 teaspoon of cayenne pepper

Preparation:

Season the slices of turkey evenly with salt and pepper on both sides. Heat up the olive oil over a medium heat. Brown the turkey meat on both sides and transfer to a plate. Set aside. Add the oil, orange zest, orange juice, cayenne and the stock in the same pan and cook until it reaches to a simmer. Return the turkey meat in the pan and baste with sauce.

Cover with lid, bring it to a boil and reduce heat to low. Simmer for 45 to 60 minutes or until the meat is tender and cooked through. If the sauce is not yet thick, cook further without the lid until the desired consistency is achieved.

Transfer the turkey meat to a serving platter, drizzle over with sauce and serve immediately.

Nutrition information per serving: Kcal: 123 Protein: 13.5g, Carbs: 16.8g, Fats: 2.8g

40. Thai beef curry

Ingredients:

2 pounds of beef chuck steak, sliced into thin strips

2 tablespoons of olive oil

2 tablespoons kaffir lime leaves, thinly sliced

1 cup unsweetened coconut milk

½ cup beef stock or water (optional)

3 tsp of sugar

1 teaspoon salt

¼ cup of Panang curry paste

Directions:

In a stew pot over medium-high heat, add 1 tablespoon of oil and fry the kaffir lime leaves briefly. Add in the curry paste, reduce to low heat and cook for about 3 minutes or until aromatic.

Add the meat and cook for 5 minutes while stirring occasionally. Stir in the stevia, and then pour in the stock and coconut milk. Briefly, stir to evenly distribute the ingredients and cover with lid. Bring it to a boil and reduce heat to low. Simmer for 30 to 35 minutes or until the beef is tender and cooked through.

Adjust taste and cook further to adjust the consistency of sauce.

Portion the beef curry into individual serving bowls or transfer into a serving bowl and serve immediately.

Nutrition information per serving: Kcal: 420 Protein: 20.5g, Carbs: 19.6g, Fats: 32.2g

Dinner Recipes

41. Grilled tuna steaks

Ingredients:

¼ cup of chopped fresh coriander leaves

3 garlic cloves, minced

2 tablespoons of lemon juice

½ cup olive oil

4 tuna steaks

½ teaspoon smoked paprika

½ teaspoon cumin, ground

½ teaspoon chili powder

Salt and black pepper

Preparation:

Add the coriander, garlic, paprika, cumin, chili powder and lemon juice in a food processor and pulse to combine. Gradually add in the oil and pulse the ingredients until a smooth mixture is achieved.

Transfer the mixture into a bowl, add the fish and gently toss to coat the fish evenly with sauce. Chill for at least 2 hours to allow the flavors to penetrate into the fish.

Remove the fish from the chiller and preheat the gas/charcoal grill. Lightly brush the grid with oil, place the fish and grill for about 3 to 4 minutes on each side.

Remove the fish from the grill, transfer to a serving plate and serve with lemon wedges or preferred sauce.

Nutrition information per serving: Kcal: 240 Protein: 53.5g, Carbs: 4g, Fats: 2g

42. Green bean burritos

Ingredients:

1 cup of cooked green beans

1 pound of lean ground beef

1 cup of cottage cheese

½ cup of chopped onions

1 tsp of ground red pepper

1 tsp of chili powder

6 whole grain tortillas

Preparation:

Cook up the meat and rinse it. Chop it into bite size pieces and put it back in the pan. Add ground red pepper, chili powder and onions. Stir well for 15 minutes. Remove from the heat.

Combine cottage cheese with green beans in a blender. Mix well for 30 seconds. Add the cheese mixture to the meat. Divide this mixture into 6 equal pieces and spread over tortillas. Wrap and serve.

Nutrition information per serving: Kcal: 310 Protein: 14.5g, Carbs: 45.2g, Fats: 8.3g

43. Egg and avocado puree

Ingredients:

4 eggs

1 cup of skim milk

½ avocado

Preparation:

Hard boil your eggs. Remove from the heat and allow it to cool. Peel and cut the eggs. Add a pinch of salt and leave in the refrigerator for about 30 minutes. Place in a blender. Cut avocado into small pieces and add to the blender. Add milk and blend for 30 minutes. This puree should be eaten right away.

Nutrition information per serving: Kcal: 205 Protein: 13.4g, Carbs: 5.7g, Fats: 13.9g

44. Walnut and strawberries salad

Ingredients:

½ cup of ground walnuts

2 cups of fresh strawberries

1 tbsp of strawberry syrup

2 tbsp of non - fat cream

1 tbsp of brown sugar

Preparation:

Wash and cut the strawberries into small pieces. Mix with ground walnuts in a bowl. In a separate bowl, combine strawberry syrup, non - fat cream and brown sugar. Beat well with a fork and use to top the salad.

Nutrition information per serving: Kcal: 131 Protein: 4.4g, Carbs: 23g, Fats: 3g

45. Ginger eggs

Ingredients:

3 eggs

2 tbsp of olive oil

1 tsp of grated ginger

1/5 tsp of pepper

¼ tsp of sea salt

Preparation:

Beat the eggs with a fork. Add ginger and pepper. Mix well and fry in olive oil for few minutes. Serve warm. Season with sea salt.

Nutrition information per serving: Kcal: 74 Protein: 2.4g, Carbs: 8.1g, Fats: 4.2g

46. Chia seeds pate

Ingredients:

½ cup of chia seeds powder

¼ cup of chia seeds

½ cup of cottage cheese

3-4 cloves of garlic

¼ cup of skim milk

1 tbsp of mustard

¼ tsp of salt

Preparation:

Chop the garlic and mix with mustard. In a large bowl, combine cottage cheese with skim milk, salt, chia seeds powder and chia seeds. Mix well and add garlic and mustard. Allow it to stand in the refrigerator for about an hour.

Nutrition information per serving: Kcal: 40 Protein: 2.6g, Carbs: 6.2g, Fats: 4.7g

47. Chicken salad recipe

Ingredients:

3 skinless, boneless chicken breast halves

1 cup of chopped lettuce

5 cherry tomatoes

2 tbsp of low fat cream

1 tbsp of olive oil

1 tsp of chopped parsley

1 tbsp of sunflower oil

1 tsp of minced chili pepper

1 tbsp of lemon juice

salt to taste

Preparation:

Cut the chicken breast halves into small cubes. Mix the sunflower oil, chopped parsley, minced chili pepper and lemon juice to make a marinade sauce. Put the chicken cubes on a baking sheet, sprinkle with chili marinade and bake at 350 degrees for about 30 minutes. Remove from the oven.

Meanwhile, mix cherry tomatoes with chopped lettuce and low fat cream. Add chicken cubes and season with salt and olive oil.

Nutrition information per serving: Kcal: 102 Protein: 9.8g, Carbs: 5.2g, Fats: 4.8g

48. Eggs and onions salad

Ingredients:

2 medium onions

4 boiled eggs

1 grated carrot

1 cup of chopped baby spinach

1 tbsp of grated fresh ginger

1 tbsp of lemon juice

1 tbsp of olive oil

1 tsp of ground turmeric

salt to taste

Preparation:

Peel and cut the onions. Salt it and leave it to stand for 15-20 minutes. Wash and squeeze, sprinkle some lemon juice over it and leave it. Meanwhile, boil the eggs for about 10 minutes, remove from heat, peel and cut into small cubes. Combine it with baby spinach, grated carrot and ginger. Add onions and season with olive oil, salt, and turmeric. Serve cold.

Nutrition information per serving: Kcal: 365 Protein: 36.4g, Carbs: 8.7g, Fats: 21.9g

49. Citrus peppered shrimps

Ingredients:

1 pound fresh large shrimps, peeled and deveined

1 organic lemon, juiced and zested

½ teaspoon black pepper, freshly ground to taste

½ teaspoon salt, or as needed to taste

½ teaspoon chili powder

1 tablespoon of extra light virgin olive oil

2 tablespoons chopped fresh parsley leaves

Preparation:

Combine together the lemon zest, lemon juice, salt, black pepper and chili powder in a large bowl and add in the shrimps. Toss to coat the shrimps with the marinade mixture and chill for at least 2 hours to marinate the shrimps.

In a wok or skillet over high heat, add the oil when the wok or skillet is very hot. Stir fry the shrimps for about 5 minutes or until opaque and thoroughly cooked.

Transfer to a serving platter, top with chopped parsley and serve with lemon wedges if desired.

Nutrition information per serving: Kcal: 142 Protein: 20.3g, Carbs: 2.8g, Fats: 6.2g

50. Kale and tomato stuffed chicken breasts

Ingredients:

4 boneless (4 ounces each), skinless chicken breasts

1 to 2 tablespoons of olive oil

½ cup soft goat's cheese

½ cup of kale, minced

¼ cup sun-dried tomatoes, chopped finely

Salt and black pepper, to taste

Preparation:

Preheat an oven to a temperature of 400°F. Lightly coat a baking dish with oil and set aside.

Add ½ cup of water into a pan, apply medium-high heat and bring to a boil. Add the kale, dried tomatoes and ½ tablespoon of oil and cook until the kale is wilted and the tomatoes have softened. Season to taste with salt and pepper and remove the pan from heat.

Slice the each breast into flat and thin pieces or flattened by a mallet. Lay the flat chicken meats on a work surface and add 1 tablespoon of cheese on the center part. Portion the kale-tomato mixture into each flat chicken meat, place them on the bottom side of the meat and season to taste with salt and pepper.

Roll the chicken upwards to cover the stuffing. Insert a toothpick on the end part of the meat to secure the stuffing. Lightly brush the top part with oil and transfer into the greased baking dish.

Bake it in the oven for about 25 minutes or until the chicken is thoroughly cooked and nicely browned. Remove from the oven and let it rest for 10 minutes before slicing and serving.

Serve warm with tomato salsa if desired.

Nutrition information per serving: Kcal: 420 Protein: 23.2g, Carbs: 23.7g, Fats: 1.7g

51. Lemon-rosemary marinated grilled chicken

Ingredients:

4 chicken breasts (4 ounce each), deboned and halved

2 tablespoons of clarified butter

1 organic lemon, juiced and zested

2 teaspoons dried rosemary leaves

2 garlic cloves, minced

1 teaspoon crushed black pepper

½ teaspoon table salt

4 slices of lemon wedges, for serving

1 tablespoon of olive oil, for coating and greasing

Preparation:

Combine together the lemon juice, lemon zest, rosemary, garlic, salt and pepper in a mixing bowl and add in the chicken. Coat the chicken evenly with the marinade mixture and chill for at least 2 hours.

Preheat the gas or charcoal grill and lightly brush the cooking grids with oil. Place the chicken on the grid and grill for about 5 to 10 minutes on each side.

Combine the ghee and marinade mixture, and brush it evenly on all sides the chicken while grilling.

When the chicken is done, remove it from the grill and let it rest for 5 minutes. Transfer to a serving platter and serve warm with lemon wedges if desired.

Nutrition information per serving: Kcal: 274 Protein: 27.2g, Carbs: 4.3g, Fats: 17.1

52. Eggs with fried vegetables and chia seeds

Ingredients:

2 eggs

3 egg whites

1 small onion

1 small carrot

1 small tomato

2 medium red peppers

1 tbsp of ground chia seeds

salt

1 tbsp of olive oil

Preparation:

Wash and pat dry the vegetables using a kitchen paper. Cut into slices or strips. Heat up the olive oil over a medium temperature and fry the vegetables for about 10 minutes, stirring constantly. Add chia seeds and mix well. You want to wait until the vegetables soften and add eggs. Fry for another 2-3 minutes. Remove from the heat and serve.

Nutrition information per serving: Kcal: 190 Protein: 15.7g, Carbs: 2g, Fats: 14.6g

53. Chicken Wings

Ingredients:

12 to 18 chicken wings

1 teaspoon ground ginger

1 tablespoon honey

2 teaspoons olive oil

1/3 cup Worcestershire Sauce

2 minced green onions

2 minced garlic cloves

Preparation:

You simply have to apply all the ingredients on the chicken wings and put them in the pot. Set the heat to low-medium and cook for about an hour. The wings should be golden brown in color indicating they have been well-cooked. You can add spices according to your liking. Serve as an appetizer with ketchup or any sauce you like.

Nutrition information per serving: Kcal: 82 Protein: 7.8g, Carbs: 1.5g, Fats: 5.8g

54. Beans and spinach

Ingredients:

1 cup of canned green beans

1 cup of chopped spinach

2 cans of tuna, without oil

1 tbsp of olive oil

1 tsp of red wine vinegar

salt to taste

1 tbsp of ground turmeric

Preparation:

Combine the green beans with chopped spinach and tuna. Season with olive oil, vinegar, and salt. Add some turmeric before serving.

Nutrition information per serving: Kcal: 318 Protein: 12.3g, Carbs: 36.7g, Fats: 17.1g

55. Light turkey lunch

Ingredients:

3 thin slices of smoked turkey breast

1 cup of lettuce

1 small tomato

1 small onion

1 red pepper

1 tbsp of lemon juice

salt to taste

Preparation:

Cut the vegetables into small pieces. Combine them with turkey breast slices and season with salt and lemon juice.

Nutrition information per serving: Kcal: 190 Protein: 15.2g, Carbs: 18.3g, Fats: 6g

56. Tuna with olives

Ingredients:

2 cups of canned tuna without oil

1 cup of chopped lettuce

1 small onion

½ cup of olives

¼ cup of chopped red pepper

1 tbsp of olive oil

salt

1 tbsp of lemon juice

Preparation:

Peel and cut the onion into small pieces. Combine it with canned tuna and chopped lettuce. Mix well. Add olives and chopped red pepper. Season with olive oil, salt, and lemon juice. Keep in the refrigerator for about 20-30 minutes.

Nutrition information per serving: Kcal: 350 Protein: 20.2g, Carbs: 21.2g, Fats: 19.7g

57. Cottage cheese with lime dressing

Ingredients:

2 cups of cottage cheese

1 large cucumber

½ cup of ground walnuts

¼ cup of lime juice

¼ cup of low fat cream

1 tsp of lime extract

1 tbsp of olive oil

¼ tsp of pepper

Preparation:

First, you want to make a lime dressing. Mix the lime juice with low fat cream, lime extract, and olive oil. Add some pepper (this part depends on your taste). Mix well and leave in the fridge for about 30 minutes. Peel and cut the cucumber into small cubes and combine with ground walnuts and cottage cheese. Pour the dressing over your salad and serve cold.

Nutrition information per serving: Kcal: 201 Protein: 18.2g, Carbs: 26.4g, Fats: 1.5g

58. Creamy lentils

Ingredients:

1 cup of canned lentil

1 small eggplant

¼ cup of low fat cream

¼ cup of lemon juice

2 tbsp of olive oil

1 tbsp of chopped parsley

1 large tomato

1 small onion

Preparation:

Peel and wash the eggplant. Cut into thin slices and combine with a low fat cream, lemon juice, and olive oil. Use an electric mixer or a blender to get a smooth mousse. Allow it to cool in the refrigerator for about 30 minutes. Meanwhile cut the vegetables into thin slices. Mix with lentil and eggplant mousse. Sprinkle with some parsley and serve.

Nutrition information per serving: Kcal: 287 Protein: 17.2g, Carbs: 30.3g, Fats: 11.7g

59. Rice with mushrooms

Ingredients:

½ cup of brown rice

2 cups of fresh bottom mushrooms

1 tbsp of oil

1 large tomato

¼ cup of fresh parsley

¼ cup of lime juice

salt

pepper

Preparation:

First, you need to cook the rice. Wash and rinse it and put in a saucepan with 1 cup of water. Stir well and bring to the boiling point. Cover the pan with a lid and cook for about 15 minutes on a low temperature. Remove from the heat and allow it to cool.

Now you want to prepare the button mushrooms. Wash and cut into similar size pieces. Heat a frying pan on a low temperature and add the oil. Add mushrooms and stir well.

Fry on a low temperature until all the mushrooms soften, or until all the water evaporates. Remove from the frying pan. Add salt and mix with rice.

Cut tomato into small cubes and combine all the ingredients with rice and mushrooms. Season with salt, pepper and lime juice. Serve warm.

Nutrition information per serving: Kcal: 324 Protein: 9.9g, Carbs: 42.8g, Fats: 15.2g

60. Cucumber with yogurt

Ingredients:

1 large cucumber

1 tsp of ground garlic

1 cup of low - fat yogurt

1 tbsp of cottage cheese

Preparation:

Peel and cut the cucumber into thin slices. Mix with yogurt, cheese, and garlic. Leave in the refrigerator for at least 30 minutes before serving. You can add some salt, but this is optional.

Nutrition information per serving: Kcal: 217 Protein: 10.7g, Carbs: 11.8g, Fats: 16.5g

61. Cilantro garlic burgers topped with parmesan

Ingredients:

2 cans of lentils, drained

3 cloves of garlic, minced

½ cup of breadcrumbs

¼ cup of parmesan cheese (freshly grated is best, but whatever you got will work)

1 egg, beaten

2 cups of water

½ cup of flour

salt and pepper to taste

Preparation:

In a medium size bowl, mash lentils with folk then mix with garlic, breadcrumbs, and cheese. Form into patties; set aside. Whisk egg and water in a bowl; flour and salt & pepper in another bowl. Coat each patty gently with flour mixture, dip into egg, then coat again with flour. Over medium-high heat in a large skillet, heat oil. Fry the burgers until lightly brown, about 2-3 minutes each side.

Serve with warm bread or in a pita with cilantro, yogurt, onion, tomatoes and whatever else you like – but this is optional!

Nutrition information per serving: Kcal: 115 Protein: 5.9g, Carbs: 28.8g, Fats: 2.1g

ADDITIONAL TITLES FROM THIS AUTHOR

70 Effective Meal Recipes to Prevent and Solve Being Overweight: Burn Fat Fast by Using Proper Dieting and Smart Nutrition

By

Joe Correa CSN

48 Acne Solving Meal Recipes: The Fast and Natural Path to Fixing Your Acne Problems in Less Than 10 Days!

By

Joe Correa CSN

41 Alzheimer's Preventing Meal Recipes: Reduce or Eliminate Your Alzheimer's Condition in 30 Days or Less!

By

Joe Correa CSN

70 Effective Breast Cancer Meal Recipes: Prevent and Fight Breast Cancer with Smart Nutrition and Powerful Foods

By

Joe Correa CSN

www.ingramcontent.com/pod-product-compliance
Lightning Source LLC
Chambersburg PA
CBHW062146020426
42334CB00020B/2534